# A Beginner's Guide to Earthquake Disaster Management

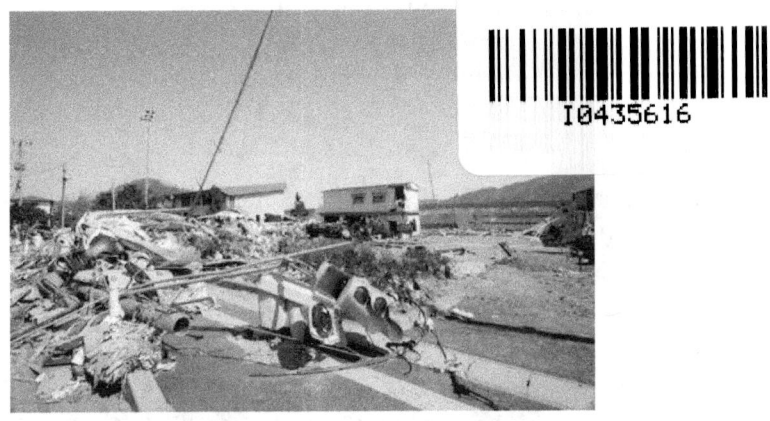

## Prepping and Survival Books

**Dueep Jyot Singh and John Davidson**

*JD-Biz Publishing*

**Disclaimer**

The information is this book is provided for informational purposes only. It is not intended to be used and medical advice or a substitute for proper medical treatment by a qualified health care provider. The information is believed to be accurate as presented based on research by the author.

The contents have not been evaluated by the U.S. Food and Drug Administration or any other Government or Health Organization and the contents in this book are not to be used to treat cure or prevent disease.

The author or publisher is not responsible for the use or safety of any diet, procedure or treatment mentioned in this book. The author or publisher is not responsible for errors or omissions that may exist.

**Warning**

The Book is for informational purposes only and before taking on any diet, treatment or medical procedure, it is recommended to consult with your primary health care provider.

Check out some of the other Healthy Gardening Series books at Amazon.com

Gardening Series on Amazon

Check out some of the other Health Learning Series books at Amazon.com

Health Learning Series on Amazon

# Table of Contents

# Introduction

Earthquakes have long been powerful natural calamities influencing the life and times of mankind down the centuries. One would not be surprised if the lost lands of Atlantis were buried under the sea because of a powerful underwater earthquake. In the same manner the Himalayan mountain range came out from under the Tethys sea millenniums ago, due to this upheaval when the tectonic plates of the land shifted and changed the topography of what is now known as the Indian subcontinent.

So is it a wonder that earthquakes have always been considered by humans down the ages to be caused due to the wrath of the gods or due to some other supernatural mysterious agency, which created and destroyed and was terrible in its intensity while it lasted.

Excavations in ancient China brought to light earthquake indicators made millenniums ago. These were frogs made up of metal, which had light round balls in their mouths. The moment the ground trembled in the vicinity, the vibrations would reach the metal, and the balls would drop down into the bowls underneath the frogs' mouths.

I have a feeling that the ancient Chinese were used to earthquakes, because as far as I know, an earthquake needed to happen, before the vibrations would register. And at that time, it would be a situation of save yourself instead of looking at the earthquake indicator.

In the same way, the Japanese also had their early warning systems to protect their lands and houses from earthquakes. Their houses were built of light materials, like bamboo and paper which would of course come down during an earthquake, but did not do much bodily harm to the inmates, when the roof literally came tumbling down. Just compare this to a house made of brick and stone, which can literally bury a family alive.

The Japanese like other Orientals are a very practical people. That is why been you that their islands were earthquake prone, so they took adequate measures to keep losses of life and property to a minimum, when these earthquakes struck. That was done millenniums ago, and those traditions are still being practiced till this day in Japan.

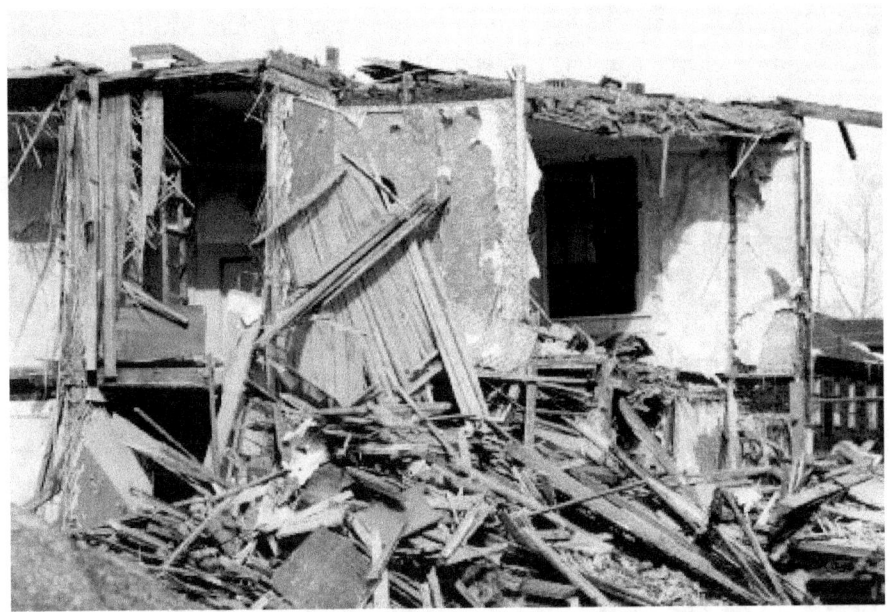

Even so, 23,000 people were killed in Kamakura in an earthquake, measuring 7.1 on the Richter scale and followed by a Tsunami and fires on 27th May, 1293.

Nevertheless, in this technologically developed 21st century world, we do not need metal frogs to give us warning of earthquakes. In fact earthquakes can be predicted in earthquake prone zones very much in advance. That makes it easier for the people to evacuate the land and property and go to much safer regions.

Earthquakes can happen either on their own, especially when the zone is earthquake prone, or they can be byproducts of other natural calamities like tsunamis and volcanic eruptions.

California – especially Los Angeles – is one earthquake prone zone, with the San Andreas Fault underground. Hollywood, of course, comes in this area. That is why the people of California are mentally geared up to face an earthquake anytime, and most of the native Californians have been subjected to tremors at least once during their lifetimes.

Believe it or not, more than 500,000 earthquakes occur every year throughout the world. The annual loss due to an earthquake in the US alone is *$200 billion.* Even though human loss has been reduced to a minimum, thanks to our early warning systems, property and human loss due to the ensuing tsunamis still reaches billions of dollars every year.

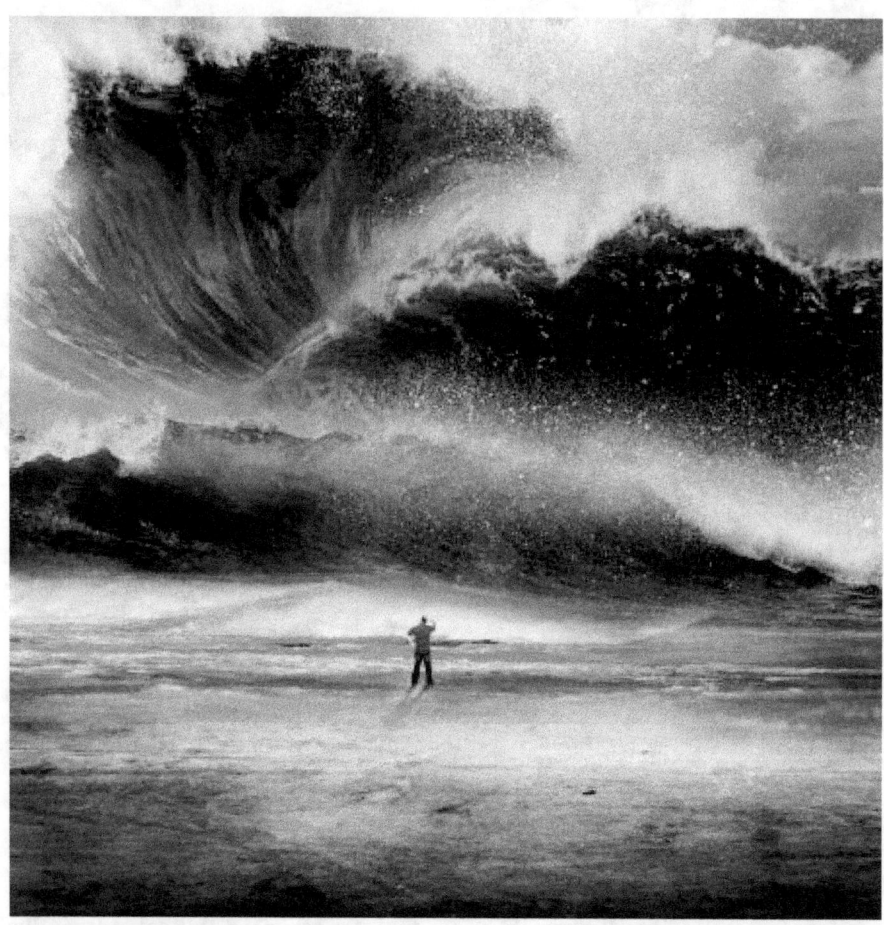

Now why is that so you may ask? That is because in many of the still developing Asian countries like India, Sri Lanka and Thailand, tsunami waves cannot be detected by early warning systems, especially when they take place under the sea in the Indian Ocean.

In 2004, my uncle happen to witness one of the 21$^{st}$ century's greatest tsunami disasters which hit the coastal areas of Thailand and other countries in the coastal region of India on the morning of 26$^{th}$ December.

People on the beach definitely did not have any tsunami warning, even though they knew that an earthquake had occurred in the vicinity. So the general populace living in the coastal areas and in places near the sea did not bother much about the possibility of a tsunami.

They also do not think that a tsunami can occur anytime in an ocean.

Uncle was having breakfast on his balcony, looking out on the sea, and wondering whether he should take a walk on the beach, which was about 10 minutes' drive away.

Suddenly he saw this huge 30 m high wall of water just rise up from the sea and in a couple of moments the beach was inundated with water. As he watched horrified and awestruck, this tsunami washed away every visible thing on the beach, including fishermen and tourists. They had absolutely no time to flee, because one of the signs of a possible tsunami did not take place. The number of casualties are not known, because most of them were locals, fishermen and tourists.

This is when the ocean recedes and exposes huge tracts of beach or land which was once under the sea. This phenomenon induces the number of people, including children to go to the beach and collect fishes which have been stranded and beached on the land. This curious investigation often has fatal results, because the sea rushes back over the beach and covers everything yet once again.[1]

It was only after this tsunami in the Indian Ocean, which does not have a communications network for warning that the United Nations decided to set up an Indian Ocean tsunami warning system in 2005. They are working on a

---

[1] Incidentally, a 10-year-old girl Tilly Smith holidaying on Maikhao beach – Phukhet – Thailand saw the receding beach and the frothy bubbles like beer on the surface of the water, and told her parents, who got the hotel and beach evacuated. About a hundred tourists were saved. This was the only beach with no fatalities during this tsunami. 200,000 people were killed in 13 countries in this terrible disaster.

global warning system, which is going to include the Pacific Ocean, Atlantic Ocean Indian Ocean and Caribbean Sea.

The Earth is undergoing more and more earthquakes every year, thanks to the shifting of the tectonic plates due to underground nuclear testing. This is one thing which scientists do not want to tell us, because their governments have forbidden them to tell the ordinary folk about the bad effect undersea and underwater and underground testing has upon the topography of the land under the surface of the earth.

That is why everybody needs to be prepared for more and more earthquakes. The delicate balance underground has already been shifted and human beings cannot repair it. Apart from that, they could not care less, because their vision is peripheral and they are bothered only about the success of underground tests.

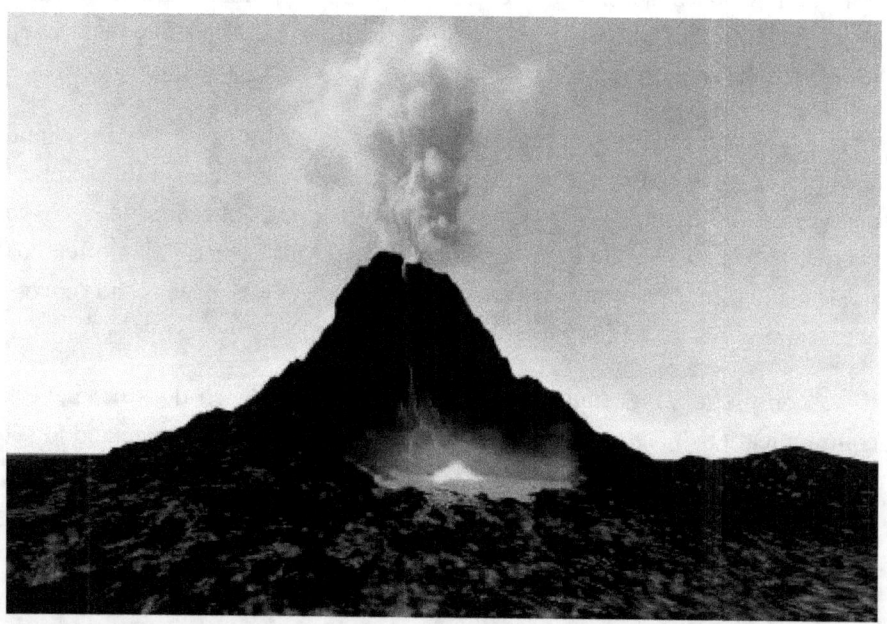

**This is the powerful force which man has disturbed due to his ignorance.**

So if you are living in an earthquake prone zone, and you also are in the vicinity of an area, where your government has done some underground testing, get ready for trouble in the future. This is not an imaginary threat, but a logical culmination and result of the harm people do when they do not think or do not want to bother about the well-being of their fellow men.

Now how did that happen? The earth is made up of many layers, which are called tectonic plates. All these layers have been shifting for millenniums, and they have a huge amount of force surrounding them. The moment these plates shift, the earth moves until the plates settle down again.

However, in the 20$^{th}$ century, this gradual shifting changed drastically, when underground testing began to be done in the 40s. And the fate of the earth underground was changed forever, with once locked plates tore apart and breaking free because of the force of the test setting free the forces of nature.

The New Madrid fault earthquake prone zone in Missouri is one of these areas. So if you are living in such a zone and are reading this book, the tips and techniques given here may come in useful sometime or the other in the near future.

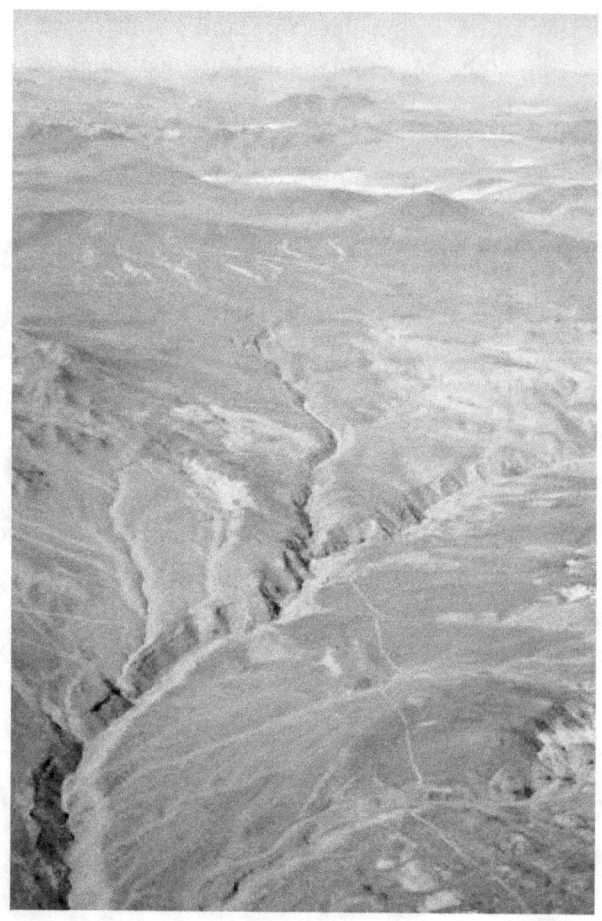

# What You Should Know about Earthquakes

If an earthquake has occurred in the area, before it is going to happen again. There is absolutely no place on our earth, which is earthquake free. However, there are areas which are not earthquake prone, because they are far away from underground testing zones and their tectonic plates have not been disturbed. Yet.

An earthquake just does not end with the earth quaking and causing lots of destruction. It is also going to bring with it, small tremors called aftershocks. These aftershocks can continue for months after the major quake. They are also going to cause more harm to already damaged buildings which were weakened due to the major quake.

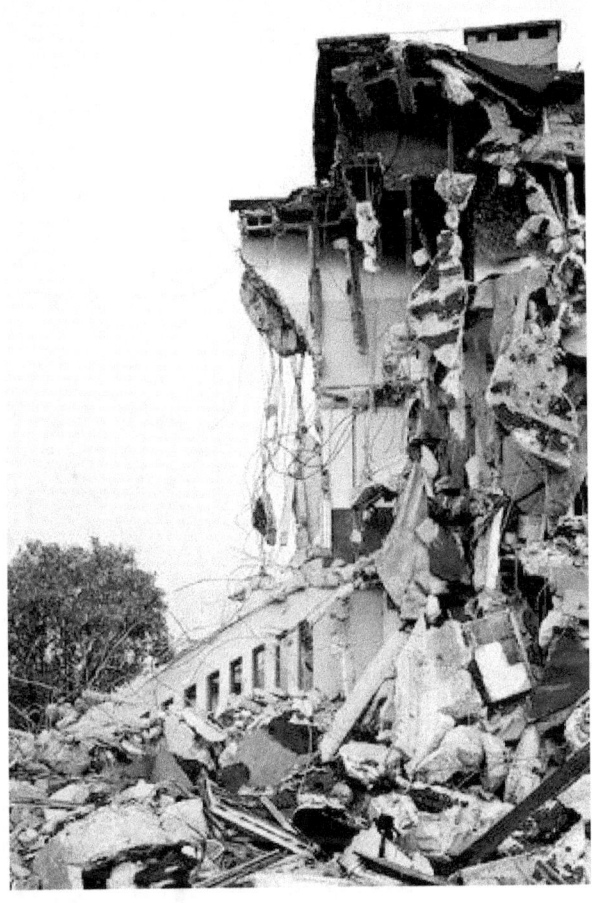

This can also work the other way around. Small earthquakes can be the precursors of another earthquake of higher magnitude.

You may want to ask the local authorities about any steps they have taken against earthquake relief, especially earthquake preparedness in your state.

People seldom get injured when the ground moves. It is the aftermath like falling walls, falling objects, and even fires which cause destruction and injuries. Many of these mishaps and tragedies can be prevented if you know how to act during an earthquake.

The moment you feel an earthquake occurring, get out from the middle of the room, and reach the corner of the wall. If you are outside, make sure that you are in an area, which is far away from any object which may fall on you.

Always be prepared for an earthquake. There might be a chance that your family members may get separated during an earthquake. That is why they should know all about a known place where they can reach or some message which they can send to assure you about their safety.

Identity discs and tags, like the ones used in the defense forces should always be carried on you, so that in case of injuries, the hospital authorities know your name, address, relatives or persons to contact in a case of emergency, and phone number.

## What Are the Aftermaths of an Earthquake

Apart from possible tsunamis, and even resultant fires, an earthquake can collapse man-made structures as well as natural structures. You are going to see a disruption of all the man-made services, including water, electricity, gas, communication and phone services.

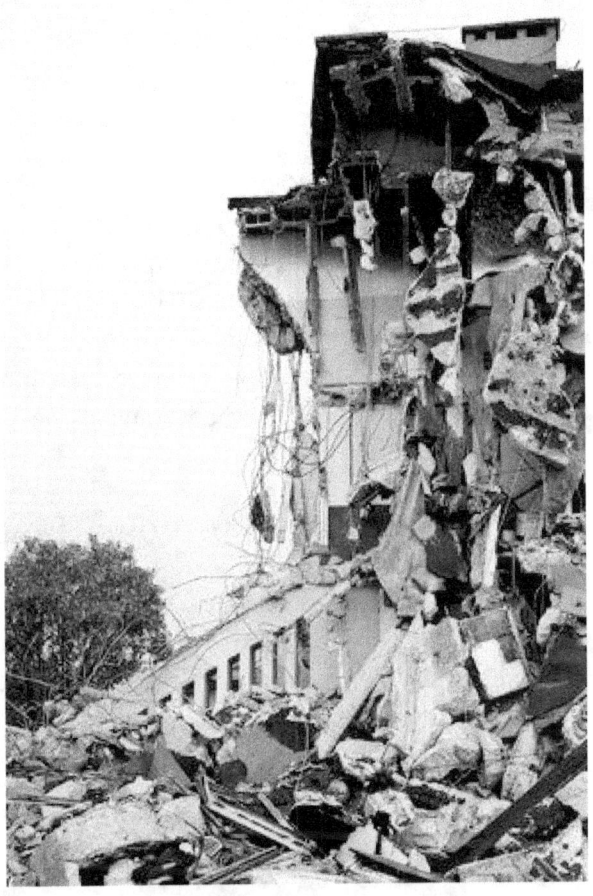

Avalanches, fires, flash floods, landslides and other natural calamities, including volcanoes can be triggered by an earthquake. That is because the natural force of underground liquid magma has been set free on the cracking of the surface of the earth and nature can go on its destructive binge freely.

Any building which has not been built on a solid space or has been built on an unstable landfill is going to collapse. That is because their foundations are not strong.

Unfortunately, earthquakes have been causing more damage in modern times because thanks to overpopulation, they normally strike areas, which are overpopulated. So apart from intensive property damage, a number of lives are lost and lots of injuries caused to the beings living there.

In 1994, an earthquake struck an area in California which was designed specifically to withstand earthquakes. Even though there was a comparatively less loss of life, $20 billion worth of property was damaged. In 1995, Kobe, which was not as prepared for earthquakes as Northridge, California, had to face property damage worth $96 billion and a loss of about 5300 people.

So this is the reason why more and more governments are concentrating on building codes and designs and building construction practices, along with teaching people how to survive during earthquakes. But it is going to take a long time to get implemented, especially in countries where people do not want to learn new practices or where the governments have laissez-faire attitudes.

## Which Are the Safe Places in Your House

Apart from the corner of the room, other safe places can be anyplace against interior walls and away from tall furniture, bookcases, and even Windows, and ceiling fans. You may also want to get under a desk or a table, which can provide security against falling objects.

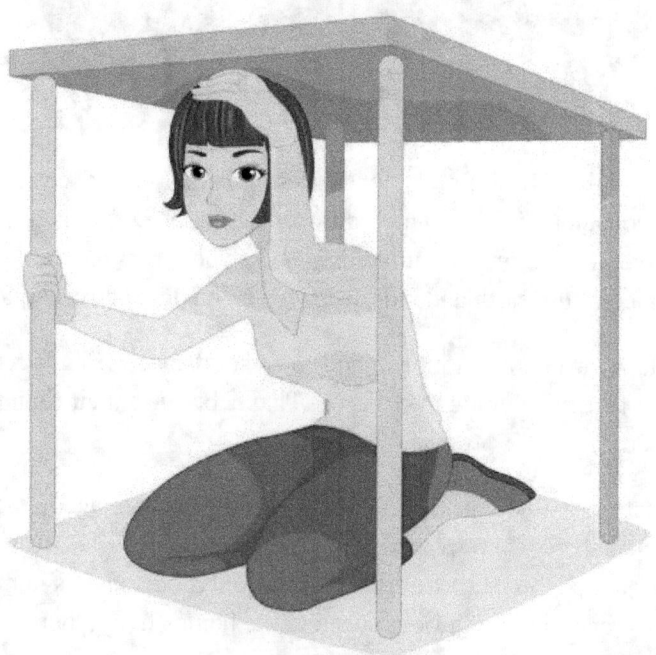

Find the easiest safe place within the couple of feet in a room, when you enter it. The further the distance you have to travel to find a safe place, the more vulnerable you are to injuries and accidents during an earthquake.

Practice how to get under a safe place – if it is the table – take cover, to protect yourself, and cover your face from injuries with your arms. A continuous practice of this procedure is going to make it automatic, when you dive for shelter during an earthquake.

Why I am suggesting that you practice is that the moment an earthquake occurs, human beings are so panic stricken, that they begin to spend time, wondering what they need to do next. However, if they know through practice what needs to be done, the mind is going to take over, and the body is going to obey.

An automatic response can make all the difference between injury and safety, life and death. Frequent practice of this dropping down, covering yourself and holding on to your shelter, is going to make this an automatic response. So try to practice this as often as possible.

See if there are and you earthquake training programs, started up by your state with professionals telling you what to do in case of such an emergency.

Practice going through these sessions with all the members of your family, so that they also know what to do in case of an earthquake. Also, make certain that they know how to respond to an earthquake, even if you are not present to guide them, when the earthquake occurs.

Stay away from windows, during an earthquake because glass is going to shatter. This is going to cause injuries.

## Fear of Earthquakes

Anxiety and fear is going to be a normal state of mind for all those people living in an earthquake zone. Some of them may have gone through earthquakes and know all about the amount of destruction they can cause. Also, this mental and emotional trauma is enough to influence their lives forever. It is possible that in recounting their experiences, they might scare other members of your family about earthquakes.

But if you discuss this phenomenon with family members, and talk about it as a natural and scientific phenomenon, this scare is going to be slowly and steadily diminished in the minds of those people who have not gone through earthquakes, but have heard about them.

## First Aid Training

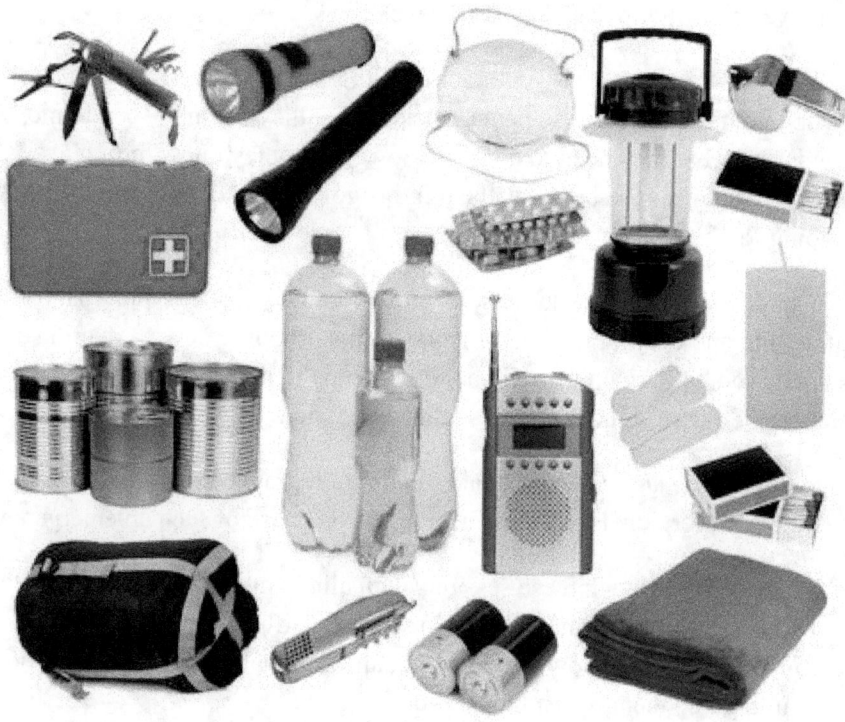

Your family members should also know all about proper first aid training, especially that given to you from Red Cross authorities in your city and state. Once adults and children get enough of confidence, that they can act in an emergency, especially when family members are injured, this is going to help a lot, against the feeling of helplessness during a natural calamity.

It is this feeling of helplessness and of what am I going to do, what can I do, what should I do, which makes a person more of a victim. However, if he has undergone some training, he knows that he will be able to cope with

---

fears and the feeling of bewilderment, terror and helplessness, during any sort of natural calamity, including earthquakes.

# Behavior of Children during Earthquakes

Only babies are totally vulnerable during earthquakes, because they depend on adults to pick them up and carry them to safety. Of course the responsibility of a baby during an earthquake has to be given to one particular responsible adult, who can be counted on not to go shrieking "Earthquake Earthquake" during such a calamity, and getting thoroughly confused.

Children need to be taught to keep calm during an earthquake. Teaching them to travel the shortest distance to the nearest safest place inside a room, or outside.

If you cannot get under a sturdy desk and hold onto the leg, sit down against the nearest interior wall and cover your face. Do not sit down against outside walls, because they are more prone to collapse.

Do not run outside, the moment an earthquake occurs, because you may get injured by pieces of construction falling from toppling buildings during an earthquake or tremor. Many casualties have occurred by people falling outside, and then getting buried under bricks, timber and roofing falling on them from the nearest toppling building.

Do not move from your safe place until the earthquake has stopped. Then check for injuries. Then check for the safety of the people around you and use your first aid practice on them, until you can get professional help. Remember, that a helping hand, especially one with first aid experience is always a boon to the overworked rescue crews after a disaster. Also, keeping busy is going to prevent you from dissolving into hysteria and shock.

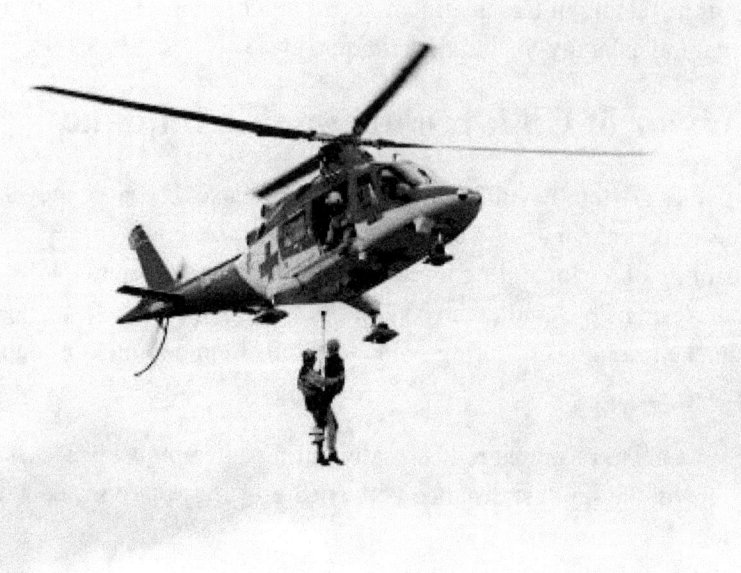

**It may take a while for the rescue teams to swing into action, so do not lose heart, and keep your morale high**

I asked a person who had gone through a bad earthquake experience about what his state of mind was, when he saw everything being destroyed around him. Remember, this was not curiosity or just hunting for cheap thrills – like that done by a TV crew, where the reporter put her microphone in the face of an earthquake victim being carried away on a stretcher and warbled in the ghastly show of sprightliness much treasured by these reporters – "you have just been rescued from an earthquake zone, how do you feel? Our viewers would like to know." That person was on the point of death. How did he feel? Struggling for life, thank you.

But then there is always some insensitive person, asking fool questions and getting in the way of serious rescue teams during any natural calamity and disaster.

Anyway, I asked him how he felt, and he said that he knew that the shock would come later, but he did what needed to be done right then, and after it was done, he had to go to the next thing, and so on, until his mind settled down.

Now, this sort of mental attitude can only be taken by a very strong-minded person, because most of us would have a tendency of figuratively diving under our nearest security blankets, and sucking our thumbs not facing reality. We would rather remain in a state of mental and physical haze and daze, because that is the only way in which we can keep reality, far away from us.

With the reality comes responsibility and most of us hate the idea that we will have to pick up our lives and carry on.

So once you are ready to go on to the next thing you need to do, after you have checked the physical, mental and emotional conditions of yourself and your family, – this includes checking shock, terror and hysteria and nipping it at the first go itself – you may want to survey the physical damage to your surroundings.

Look out for hazards while moving around carefully. Be prepared for more aftershocks. Fires are a hazard which can occur after an earthquake, especially when gas lines are broken or electric lines have been damaged. Also, sparks from previously lit fires can also start other fires, especially when an earthquake brings an inflammable object near to a source of fire.

Never use an elevator during or after an earthquake. If you are exiting a building, always use the stairs.

If an earthquake occurs at night, and you are in bed, protect your head with the pillow, after you have rolled away from under the ceiling fan. This is one of the hazards which can harm you, especially if your bed is directly underneath it.

If you are outside in the open air, when an earthquake occurs, do not take the shelter of a building, by sitting down in the shelter of its outer wall. You are just asking to be covered and injured by falling debris, if you do so.

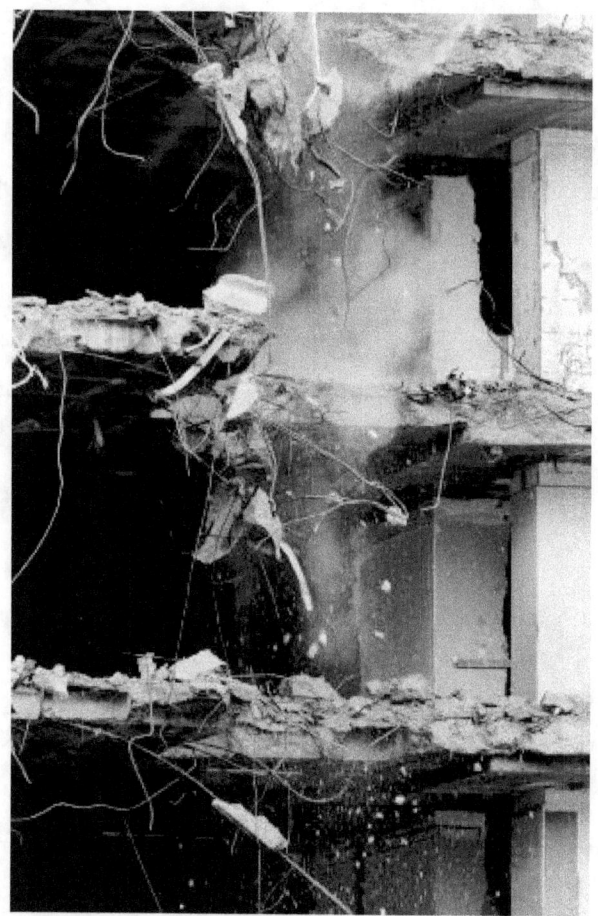

Move as far away as you can from a building, and go out in an open area. Keep away from streetlights, trees, and any other building constructions or power lines.

Crouch down to ground level and protect your head with your arms.

## Emergency Earthquake Disaster Kit

I have a basic emergency and earthquake disaster kit right next to my bed, which consists of basic supplies. These include clothes, medicines, an extra pair of shoes and socks, and a larger backpack for each family member which includes these essential items, in case we have to evacuate.

Remember that in case of an earthquake, you may need to have enough of supplies to last you anywhere between 48 hours to 72 days, depending on how fast rescue teams can get to you.

# Home

In your home, you need to have these supplies ready at hand.

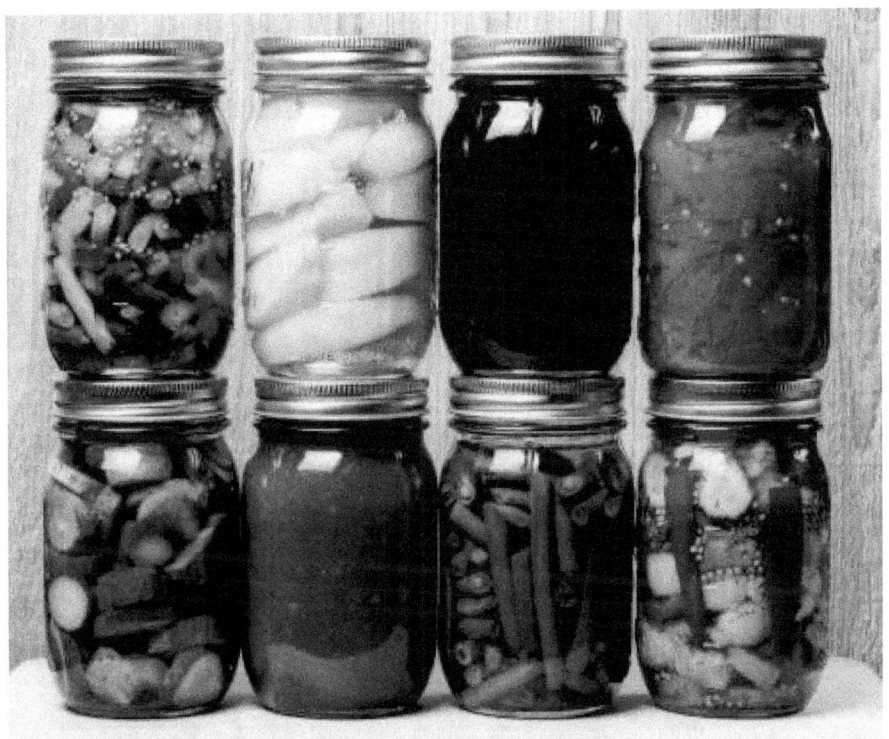

**Plenty of preserved food ready at hand is always a positive mental and physical support to you during a catastrophe.**

Plenty of canned food, and nonperishable food, which can help feed your family. Every family member needs to have 1 gallon of fresh water per day, so make sure that there are ready with supplies of water ready at hand. I would suggest having gallon cartons full of water. These cartons should be replaced every six months.

Add eight drops of liquid bleach, which is unscented, to every gallon of water, when you start storing it. Keep replacing this water periodically. If there is a fungal growth at the bottom of the container, remove the water, clean the container, and refill it with fresh water.

Your pets come in "family". So make sure that there are enough food supplies and water for your pets too.

Necessary tools include manual bottle openers and can openers, a reliable lighter to light fire, candles and matches and adequate fuel supplies to keep you supplied with warmth and light, with the help of a paraffin or kerosene stove.

Items which keep your family warm, especially when there is no electricity will include plenty of blankets and sleeping bags.

A good first aid kit is going to include bandages, medicines, thermometer, antibiotics and personal hygiene and sanitary items. Also, list of your personal medical devices, including pacemaker, diabetes control kit and other health related items should be listed in a list on your first aid kit box and pasted on the cover. Also, the name of your family doctor, his contact number and the number of your nearest hospital and ambulance.

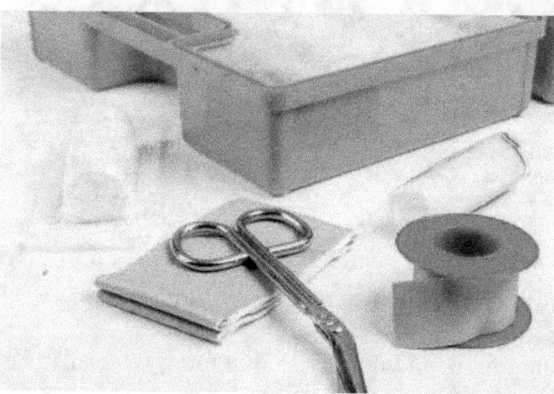

A battery-operated portable radio is excellent for you to get the latest news and bulletins. These broadcasts will keep you informed about the situation in the disaster area.

Also, keep extra pairs of eyeglasses and contact lenses near you. Also, an extra pair of dentures, if you use them.

Each family member should have a set of house keys and car keys with him on a keychain. That is, if you need to evacuate your house and drive away in your car. That is so that everybody in the family can come back to the house after it has been declared safe by the authorities.

You should also have easy access to cash, credit cards and small change in case you need money right now.

Keep water purification tablets and pellets near you, because you do not know about the state of water contamination, when the water supply gets regularized after an earthquake.

Have plenty of eating utensils, especially disposable ones near at hand. These can include plastic plates and paper plates and cutlery.

If there are elders in your family, babies and disabled people, make sure that their medications and their food items are stocked near at hand and easily accessible. They should also be replaced regularly, especially if you are stocking canned baby food in bottles and tins.

Keep a good supply of sharp knives and razor blades with you both for your safety and for use.

A good multipurpose tool, along with lots of nails and a hammer will always come in useful. Make sure that these tools are manual tools, because you are not certain whether you will have a continuous supply of electricity after an earthquake.

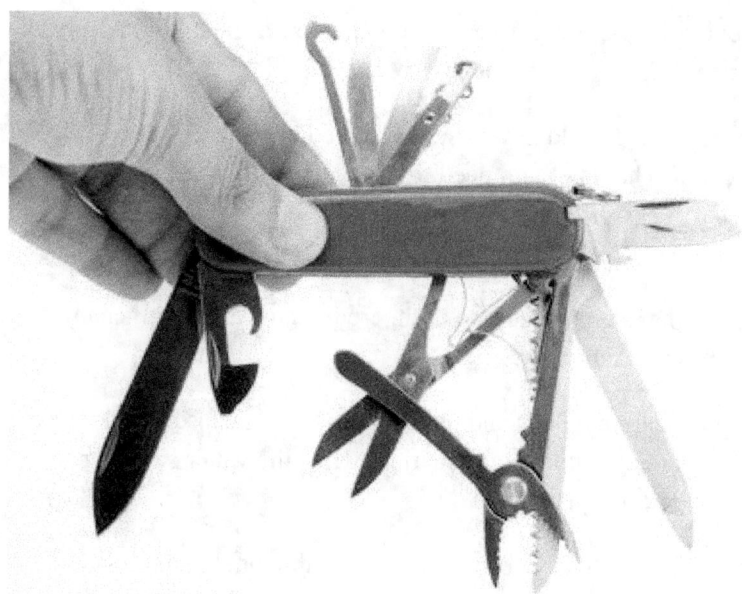

**A multipurpose Swiss knife is excellent, but I have one which includes a hammer, screwdriver, wire cutter and pliers. Look for it online or in your nearest store.[2]**

A multipurpose tool kit like this one in this URL looks interesting.

http://www.ebay.com/itm/Multi-Purpose-Tool-Kit-Outdoors-Hunting-Emergancy-/260722147900?pt=LH_DefaultDomain_0&hash=item3cb440423c

Along with this, you need plenty of candles and other sources of light along with a good flint lighter, lots of matches and also light sticks, which do not need to work on electricity.

---

[2] http://www.ebay.in/itm/10-1-MULTI-UTILITY-HAMMER-TOOL-KIT-ArmY-Knife-Screw-driver-blade-PURPOSE-/271111155375?pt=IN_Kitchenware_Dining_Bar&hash=item3f1f7beeaf

Made in China. Sold in India. Around $7-$8. Look on your country's eBay site for this item at bargain prices and free shipping.

Work gloves are going to come in handy to protect your hands, especially when you are rummaging through the debris in case portions of your house have been damaged during the earthquake.

Have plenty of wire and rope at hand. Along with that, you may need a shovel, saw and ax. A crowbar can open up  bent and twisted parts of the building.

Keep lots of sacks, as well as small and large polythene and plastic bags handy. You never know when you may need them to store items.

Needles, thread and Needles threader, along with a good pair of scissors is one thing people do not put in their survival kit. But Mother Robinson in the Swiss Family Robinson had Needles and thread in her magic purse, which served the needs of her family of four sons and husband for 14 years.

Of course, that particular book may be a favorite of children, but it is pure muddleheaded fiction with ostriches and zebras in the same territorial zone as tigers. But in reality, you need to have a number of these little items with you, because you do not know when you need them.

Also, you need a good working compass, along with plenty of road maps in your home, in the survival kit bag and also the same items in the kit bag in your car.

Have plenty of writing materials, along with paper and pens, right at hand because you never know when you will need to write a note.

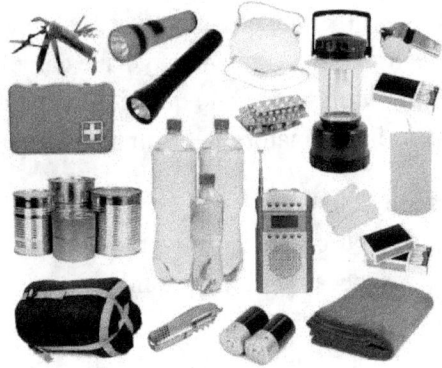

Have a bottle opener, bottled water, energy giving food, change of clothing, – depending on the weather – flashlight, transistor radio, fresh batteries, sleeping bag, blankets and a first aid box.

# Extinguishers for Electric Fires

As fire is one of the common hazards faced by people who have just suffered the aftermath of an earthquake, I asked one of my Red Cross friends, whether an electrical fire could be extinguished by a fire extinguisher, and he told me that yes, there are category C fire extinguishers, available, which do not conduct electricity.

This is because I know that most of the electric fires which occur during a calamity take place due to short-circuits.

This is when you need to have immediate access to a C category electric fire extinguisher.

Remember that only the fire department can take care of a raging fire. A fire extinguisher is that best a temporary measure to stop or dowse a limited fire and preventing it from growing.

The C category fire extinguishers found in America come under the label of BC and ABC. You also know them as dry fire extinguishers.

So, look for any extinguisher, which has a C Mark on its label. It means that it is not going to conduct electricity.

BC can be said to be bicarbonate non-electricity conducting extinguisher. These are best for electrical fires. Others may have carbon dioxide. Use them on electrical fires, when there is no question of the fire flaring up due to the presence of more inflammatory items in the vicinity.

ABC extinguishers are best, because they can be used to extinguish both conventional fires and electric fires. However, they leave a sticky residue on the electric compliments, because they are a mixture of carbon dioxide and other fireproofing materials like Mono ammonium phosphate. This is yellowish in color and the residue is clearly visible.

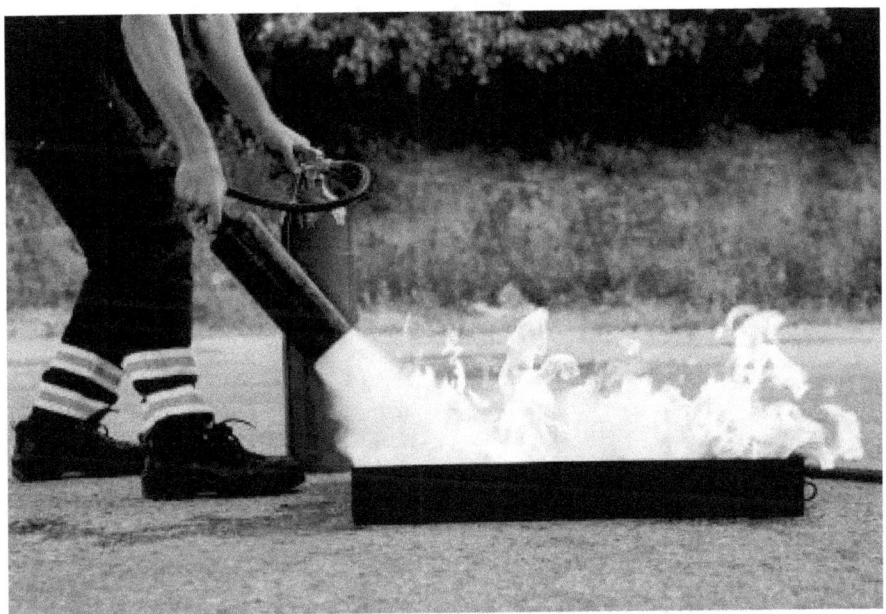

Teach your family members how to use a fire extinguisher. Get it serviced regularly and **refilled every six months.**

I am asking you this, because I believe I am the only person in the world who has had her office, literally burnt out from under her *twice* in her lifetime. [Once may be just chance, but twice is sheer pushing your luck.] And all this was due to electrical fires.

The first time we managed to escape by climbing to a nearby office building's roof, because there was *no fire extinguisher around*, the stairwell was well lit and there was no way out except try to escape from the roof. The management did not consider it necessary to invest in fire extinguishers, because hey, there was no chance of a fire occurring in their buildings. And that particular city did not bother much about fire escapes and rules and regulations regarding fire safety in buildings.

The next time round, when the fire started seeping in on our fourth floor office, we grabbed the fire extinguisher and pressed the handle. No go. **It had not been refilled and re-serviced.**

All of us escaped by breaking two of the closed windows *[cover your fist with a piece of cloth to protect it from the glass, and then smash the pane]* and wriggling out to safety. We then used the fire escape of that building – ours did not have one – to get to the ground, and safety.

 Needless to say, I resigned both these jobs as soon as I recover from smoke inhalation because I was not going to go back to places where the top management was not concerned about the safety of their employees and left them to fend for themselves in cases of fire.[3]

# Items for Your Car

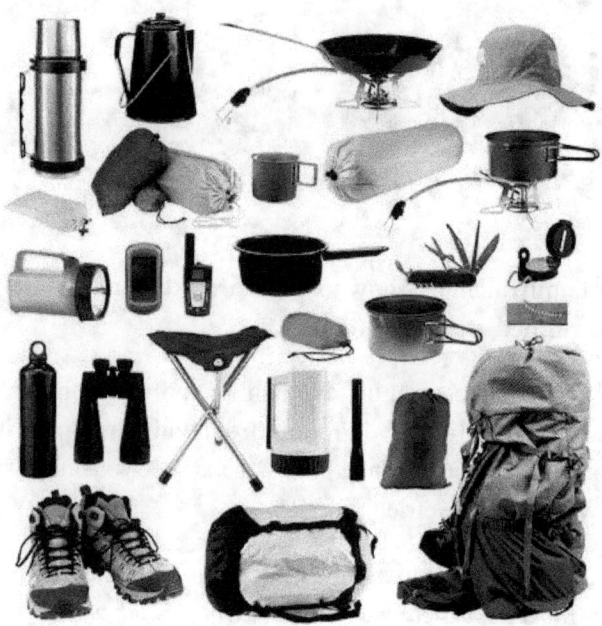

---

**These items are excellent for a trip. These are also excellent for survival kits.**

An earthquake survival kit for your car is going to include blankets for your car as well as a thermos full of hot liquids. Keep a lighter handy. Also, lots of candles. Also, a flashlight, which works, along with extra batteries for signaling purposes and for lighting purposes.

A radio, which is battery powered is essential so that you can have easy access to bulletins and news.

Your car pack should have granola, energy bars, raisins and dried fruit.

Extra clothing is always useful along with raincoats, good walking shoes and socks.

# Readying your house for An Earthquake

If your house is an earthquake zone, you may want to look at the building norms in the city, which maintain proper construction specifications. Along with this, you can prepare your interior to withstand an earthquake, by bolting all the heavy movable furniture to the wall, by bracing or anchoring with wall studs.

Anything which can fall, is going to fall during an earthquake. So secure it like your TV, book cabinets, computer, books, etc.. Also, be sure that you are not around them, when there is an earthquake, because there is a chance of those items falling on you and causing injury.

Heavy objects in your display cabinets should be displayed on the lower shelves. These will cause less chances of potential damage and injury when they fall.

In the same manner, all the fragile items, and breakable items like bottled goods, glass showpieces, porcelain, China and other items should be placed in closed cabinets, on low shelves. Latch these securely. This is going to prevent the cabinet from flying open during an earthquake and spreading its contained items all over the floor.

The bottom shelves can also be used to store flammable products, chemical products, pesticides, cleaners, and detergents.

Your bedroom should not have a heavy picture overhanging the wall over your bed. Just imagine that heavy frame falling down on your head while you are asleep.

Someone asked me why the walls in my house did not have heavy items like mirrors and pictures hanging on them, and I told them that I lived in an earthquake zone. The only thing I need to worry about, falling in these rooms – apart from the roof, of course – are the ceiling fans! Everything else is locked and bolted down. Even the light fixtures and the curtain pelmets overhead were braced so that they did not fall and cause injury.

In the kitchen and in the bathrooms, make sure that the hot water heater and geysers are strapped properly to the wall. The water heater in your kitchen may be the best and only available source of water for you to drink during an earthquake, because naturally during a calamity, you boil water before drinking it. This is to prevent you from falling sick due to waterborne diseases.

The pipe fittings should be flexible. This prevents water leaks and gas leaks. They also are less prone to break.

If there are any deep cracks in your house building foundations, on the roof, and on the outer walls, get an experienced structural expert and architect to give you the best advice on how to get this repaired. As the strength of the chain depends on its weakest link, a weak foundation means that your house is going to be more vulnerable to an earthquake and is going to be the first one to give away in the neighborhood, during any occurring tremor.

## Building Codes and Standards

An architect, while designing a house for an acquaintance suggested that the house was bolted to the foundation that would prevent it from sliding off from the foundation, and getting destroyed. So if you are intent on building a house, get an architectural plan, which includes bolting of the house to the foundation. The previously referred to Northfield, California experiment must have had buildings bolted to the foundations to keep damage to the minimum.

Remember that each territory according to its location and its proximity to a seismic zone has different building standards and codes to protect the occupants as well as property. Learn about these standards and use them when building your house.

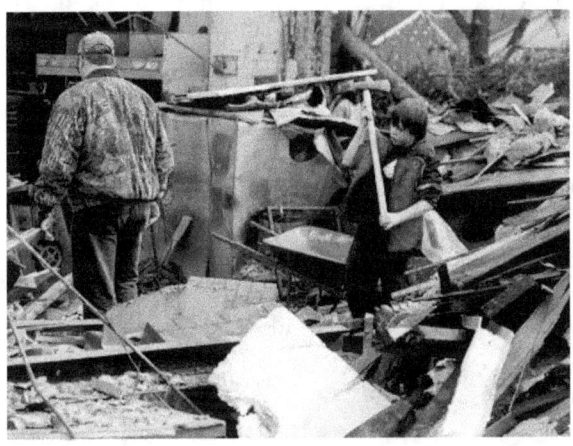

There are still plenty of places in the world, where the community and the local authorities have a laissez-faire, or ostrich attitude towards natural disasters. The attitude is that – let a calamity happen, and then we are going to tackle it. Why bother about trouble, until trouble troubles us? This all too very common and prevalent state of mind has absolutely no place in the 21$^{st}$ century.

It depends on the citizens to ask the authorities and the community to develop proper and stronger codes and standards for building and development of properties. How strong a level of an earthquake can be withstood by a structure? I went to our state's building and town planning department and asked this question of a senior officer. In return, I received a look redolent of "Huh, what are you talking about?" I was astonished and shocked at her ignorance.

She knew absolutely nothing about building requirements, which took minimum earthquake shock codes in view. She just saw the designs and passed them, and as long as they did not infringe on the city's *not more than two stories high* standard, the designs were acceptable.

My city is in an earthquake zone. There are mountain ranges nearby, and during the last year, we have been subject to three earthquakes. But nobody wants to bother about building codes. One knows what is going to happen during a major earthquake here. They are going to shriek for aid from the Central government, and then hope that somebody else is going to give them aid in the rebuilding of the city and planning it again. That is because everyone has the attitude of what is going to be is going to be, and nobody can prevent it.

Do not let that happen to your city. Get your local newspaper to publish a daily section on earthquakes, and the emergency numbers to contact, including hospitals, the Red Cross, and emergency service offices to give aid during a catastrophe.

Get an experienced team together – along with the Red Cross services, the Rotary club and other important clubs in the city – and talk about emergency services and training sessions, including drill sessions for earthquake safety and first aid.

You may want to get the public utility services officials to talk on the local radio about how to switch off the electricity, water, and gas from the main during an earthquake to prevent accidents.

## On the Road during an Earthquake

If you are on the road, and an earthquake occurs, pull over to an open location, away from trees, hoardings, power lines, street signs and buildings. Stop your vehicle, and stay in it, with your seatbelts still on, until the tremors stop.

Your vehicle is going to protect you from objects falling from above, so do not get out of it. Do not drive over bridges after the earthquake has stopped and proceed carefully, on the lookout for cracks on the road.

If you are in a mountainous area, be on the lookout for landslides as well as rock falls and avalanches. These are going to occur, whenever there is a tremor in the mountains.

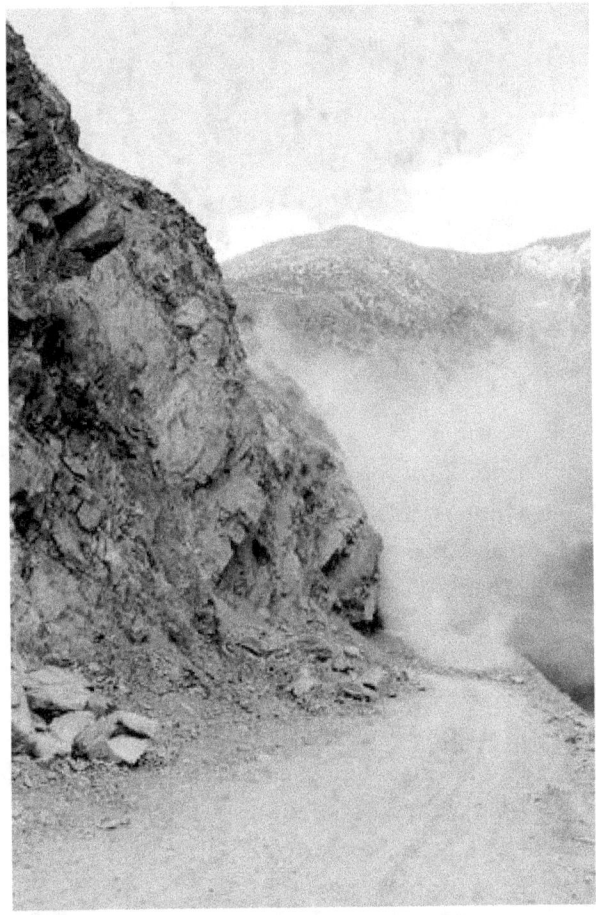

Landslides and avalanches are aftermaths of earthquakes

# Evacuation of your house

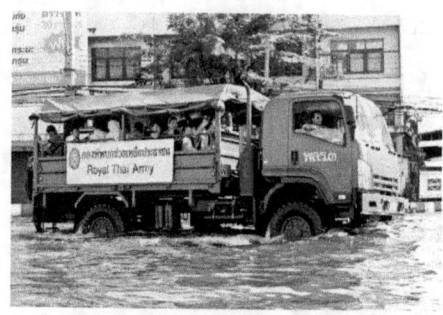

**It is more sensible to evacuate an area, especially when there is a chance of a tsunami rather than put your life in jeopardy thinking that it cannot happen.**

If you have got an earthquake warning, and have been told by authorities to evacuate your house, pick up your survival kit bag, put on a full length sleeved shirt, loose fitting pants, sturdy shoes, work gloves, and something to protect your head and then get out of the house. These clothing items will help protect your body from superficial scratches and possible injuries from broken items.

911 are going to swing into action, after an earthquake. But with your first aid training, you can start some positive work on your own, and help people who are injured. Do not deliberately put yourself in danger, by doing something reckless. People were injured seriously should not be moved by you, unless you are a trained medical expert and know how to treat head wounds, and wounds in the back.

I know about a person who met with a rather bad road accident. She had a head injury and her spinal cord was injured too. Some do-gooders, too anxious to get their names in the local paper immediately came rushing there and tried to pull her out from under the car. They broke her spinal cord while trying to drag her out because they would not be bothered to wait for the paramedics.

Unfortunately, this is what is being taught to many people during first aid lessons. Get a patient out of an accident zone, especially a car, as soon as possible. That is our first instinct. But most of us do more harm than good. There is no thin line between should we or should not we, when confronted with such a situation. But if you have experience paramedics nearby, leave the rescue in their expert hands.

In the meantime, it is much better for you to fight fires and helping in the removal of debris, instead of rescuing people from underneath buildings. The 1906 San Francisco earthquake was followed by a number of fires, which caused more damage to the city than the earthquake did. So, look at all your presently available resources and stop fires.

Do not live in your home, if it is unsafe. Get your family out to a safer place. Also, do not go inspecting it, right after an earthquake see the damage, because you may be caught or trapped under parts of your damaged home, giving way.

Use a battery-powered flashlight to inspect the interior of your home, after the authorities have declared it danger free. Inspecting it with candles or kerosene lamps and lanterns may cause accidents, if there are inflammable items in the vicinity. And most important of all, no smoking inside a damaged building, however much your stressed out and tense nerves may need that coffin nail. This can also cause a fire.

While inspecting a damaged building, keep away from wires and also gas pipes. If you smell gas or hear hissing, leave the building immediately because there is a gas leak somewhere. Turn off the gas supply in the building and call your gas company to send an experienced professional. He is going to tackle this problem. This professional is also going to turn the gas on, if you turned it off yourself.

In the same manner, the electric system is going to include damaged wires, and frayed wires and circuits. If you see any sparks, turn off the electricity from the circuit breaker or from your main fuse box. Do not approach the circuit breaker, if you have to pass through water. Instead, get a professional electrician to do this work for you.

The water supply is going to be contaminated, because you do not know whether the sewage lines are intact or not. So make sure that the drinking water which you drink has been taken from your water storage supplies or has been boiled properly and filtered before drinking. You can also get water from ice cubes which have been melted.

Do not go using telephones, unless absolutely necessary. That is because during calamity is, the lines are overloaded, and more emergency calls with a higher priority over your call need to get through faster. You may use your cell phone, if the batteries are working. That means you need to invest in a good cell phone, which does not need a battery recharge every 24 hours! Nokia and Samsung telephones are well known to have a longer battery life.

# Conclusion

The attitude of *this cannot happen to me*, especially in matters of fire, floods and earthquakes is not one which you can take in the 21ˢᵗ century. This is the century of continuous natural disasters, thanks to human depredation of the earth's resources and interfering with the natural topographical and environmental structure of the earth. And that is why he has set off a powerful force, which he cannot control. All he can do is try to control the aftereffects of these calamities as far as he can, and that includes these tips and techniques given in this book.

You may want to learn more about survival tactics and other disaster related management tips and techniques in more of my books available on this link –

Live Long and Prosper!

http://www.amazon.com/s/ref=nb_sb_noss?url=search-alias%3Daps&field-keywords=john+davidson+prepping+and+survival&rh=i%3Aaps%2Ck%3A john+davidson+prepping+and+survival

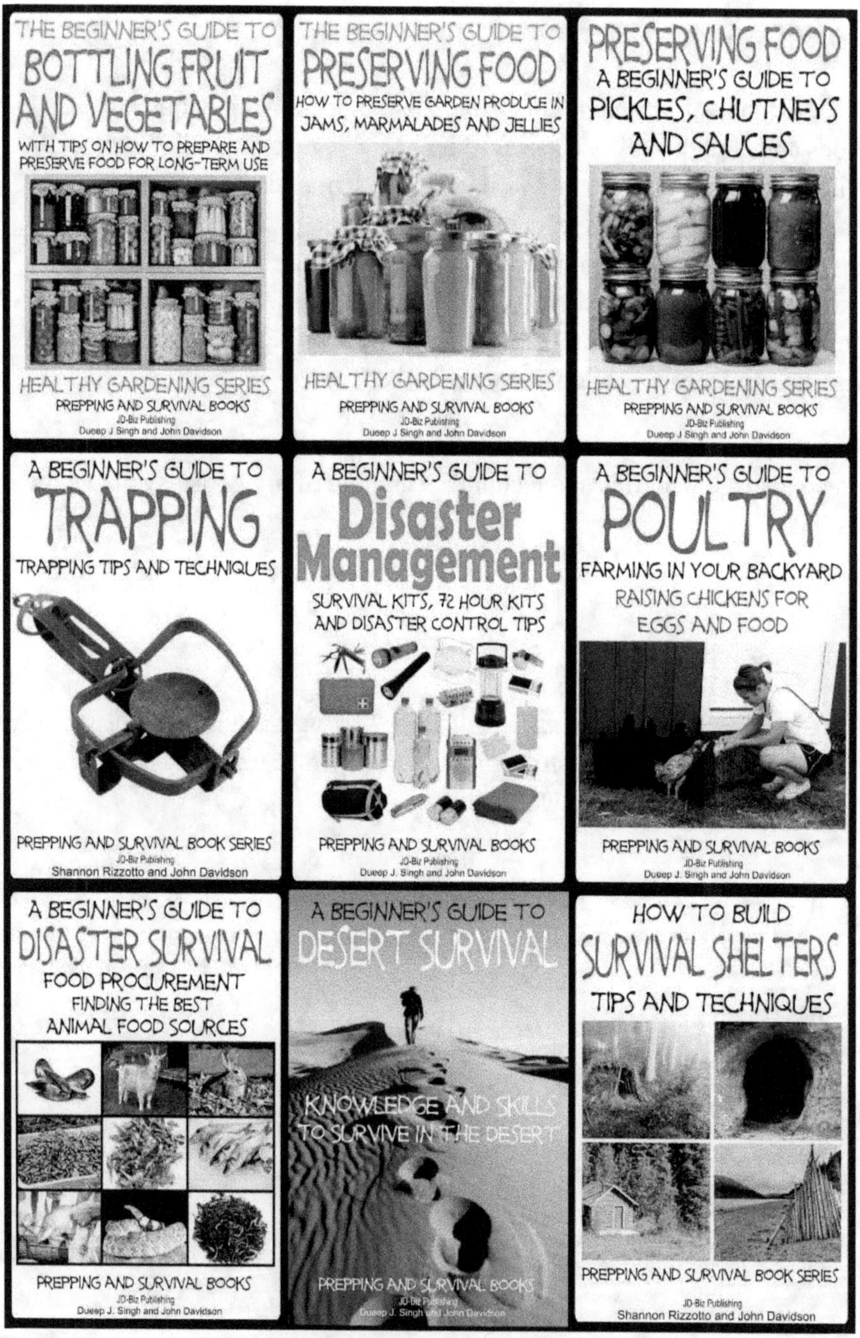

THE BEGINNER'S GUIDE TO
**BOTTLING FRUIT AND VEGETABLES**
WITH TIPS ON HOW TO PREPARE AND
PRESERVE FOOD FOR LONG-TERM USE

HEALTHY GARDENING SERIES
PREPPING AND SURVIVAL BOOKS
JD-Biz Publishing
Dueep J Singh and John Davidson

THE BEGINNER'S GUIDE TO
**PRESERVING FOOD**
HOW TO PRESERVE GARDEN PRODUCE IN
JAMS, MARMALADES AND JELLIES

HEALTHY GARDENING SERIES
PREPPING AND SURVIVAL BOOKS
JD-Biz Publishing
Dueep J Singh and John Davidson

**PRESERVING FOOD**
A BEGINNER'S GUIDE TO
PICKLES, CHUTNEYS AND SAUCES

HEALTHY GARDENING SERIES
PREPPING AND SURVIVAL BOOKS
JD-Biz Publishing
Dueep J Singh and John Davidson

A BEGINNER'S GUIDE TO
**TRAPPING**
TRAPPING TIPS AND TECHNIQUES

PREPPING AND SURVIVAL BOOK SERIES
JD-Biz Publishing
Shannon Rizzotto and John Davidson

A BEGINNER'S GUIDE TO
**Disaster Management**
SURVIVAL KITS, 72 HOUR KITS
AND DISASTER CONTROL TIPS

PREPPING AND SURVIVAL BOOKS
JD-Biz Publishing
Dueep J. Singh and John Davidson

A BEGINNER'S GUIDE TO
**POULTRY**
FARMING IN YOUR BACKYARD
RAISING CHICKENS FOR
EGGS AND FOOD

PREPPING AND SURVIVAL BOOKS
JD-Biz Publishing
Dueep J. Singh and John Davidson

A BEGINNER'S GUIDE TO
**DISASTER SURVIVAL**
FOOD PROCUREMENT
FINDING THE BEST
ANIMAL FOOD SOURCES

PREPPING AND SURVIVAL BOOKS
JD-Biz Publishing
Dueep J. Singh and John Davidson

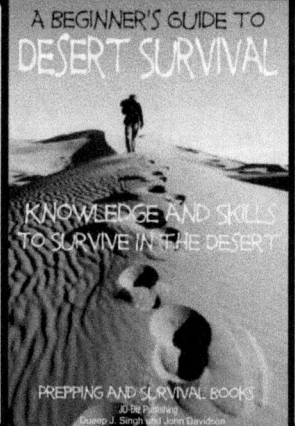

A BEGINNER'S GUIDE TO
**DESERT SURVIVAL**
KNOWLEDGE AND SKILLS
TO SURVIVE IN THE DESERT

PREPPING AND SURVIVAL BOOKS
JD-Biz Publishing
Dueep J. Singh and John Davidson

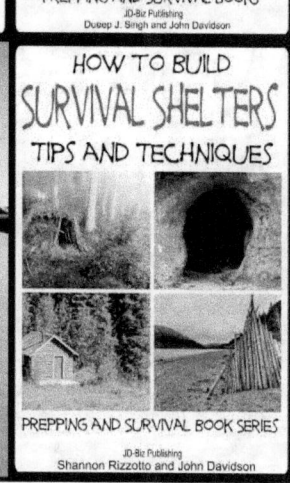

HOW TO BUILD
**SURVIVAL SHELTERS**
TIPS AND TECHNIQUES

PREPPING AND SURVIVAL BOOK SERIES
JD-Biz Publishing
Shannon Rizzotto and John Davidson

# Author Bio-

**Dueep Jyot Singh** is a Management and IT Professional who managed to gather Postgraduate qualifications in Management and English and Degrees in Science, French and Education while pursuing different enjoyable career options like being an hospital administrator, IT,SEO and HRD Database Manager/ trainer, movie , radio and TV scriptwriter, theatre artiste and public speaker, lecturer in French, Marketing and Advertising, ex-Editor of Hearts On Fire (now known as Solstice) Books Missouri USA, advice columnist and cartoonist, publisher and Aviation School trainer, ex-moderator on Medico.in, banker, student councilor ,travelogue writer … among other things!

One fine morning, she decided that she had enough of killing herself by Degrees and went back to her first love -- writing. It's more enjoyable! She already has 48 published academic and 14 fiction- in- different- genre books under her belt.

When she is not designing websites or making Graphic design illustrations for clients , she is browsing through old bookshops hunting for treasures, of which she has an enviable collection – including R.L. Stevenson, O.Henry, Dornford Yates, Maurice Walsh, De Maupassant, Victor Hugo, Sapper, C.N. Williamson, "Bartimeus" and the crown of her collection- Dickens "The Old Curiosity Shop," and so on… Just call her "Renaissance Woman" ) - collecting herbal remedies, acting like Universal Helping Hand/Agony Aunt, or escaping to her dear mountains for a bit of exploring, collecting herbs and plants and trekking.

## Our books are available at

1. Amazon.com
2. Barnes and Noble
3. Itunes
4. Kobo
5. Smashwords
6. Google Play Books

Check out some of the other JD-Biz Publishing books

Gardening Series on Amazon

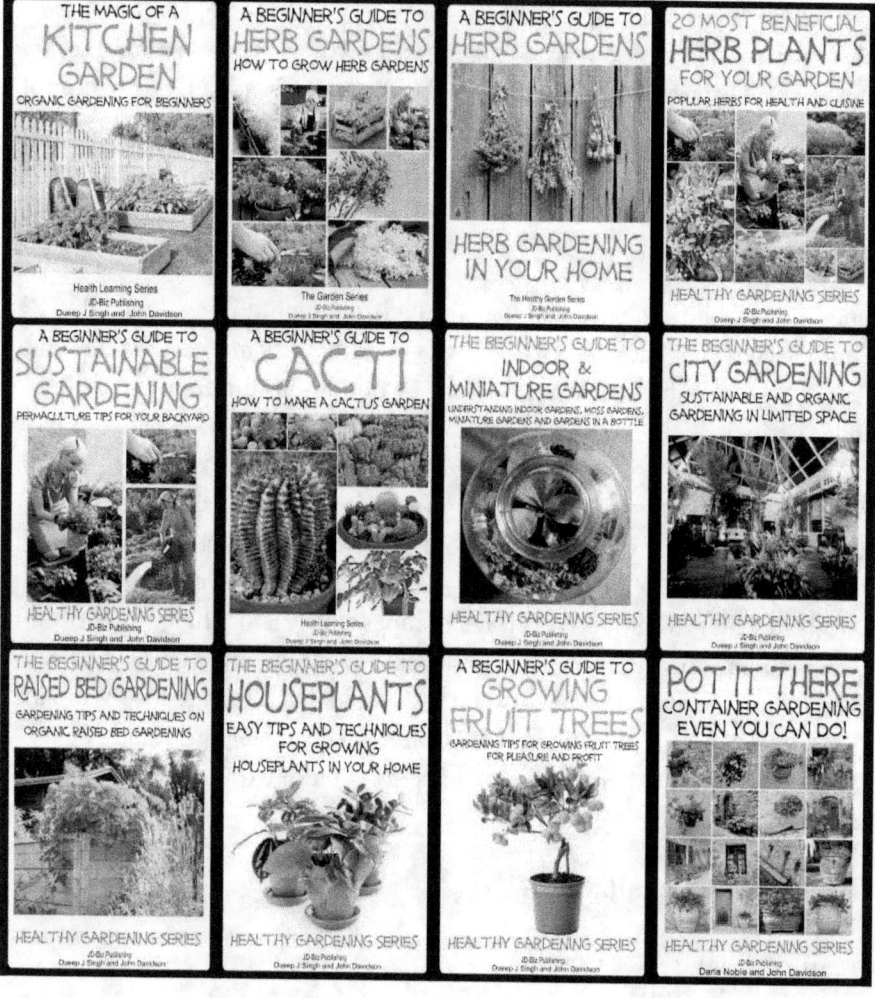

# Health Learning Series

# Country Life Books

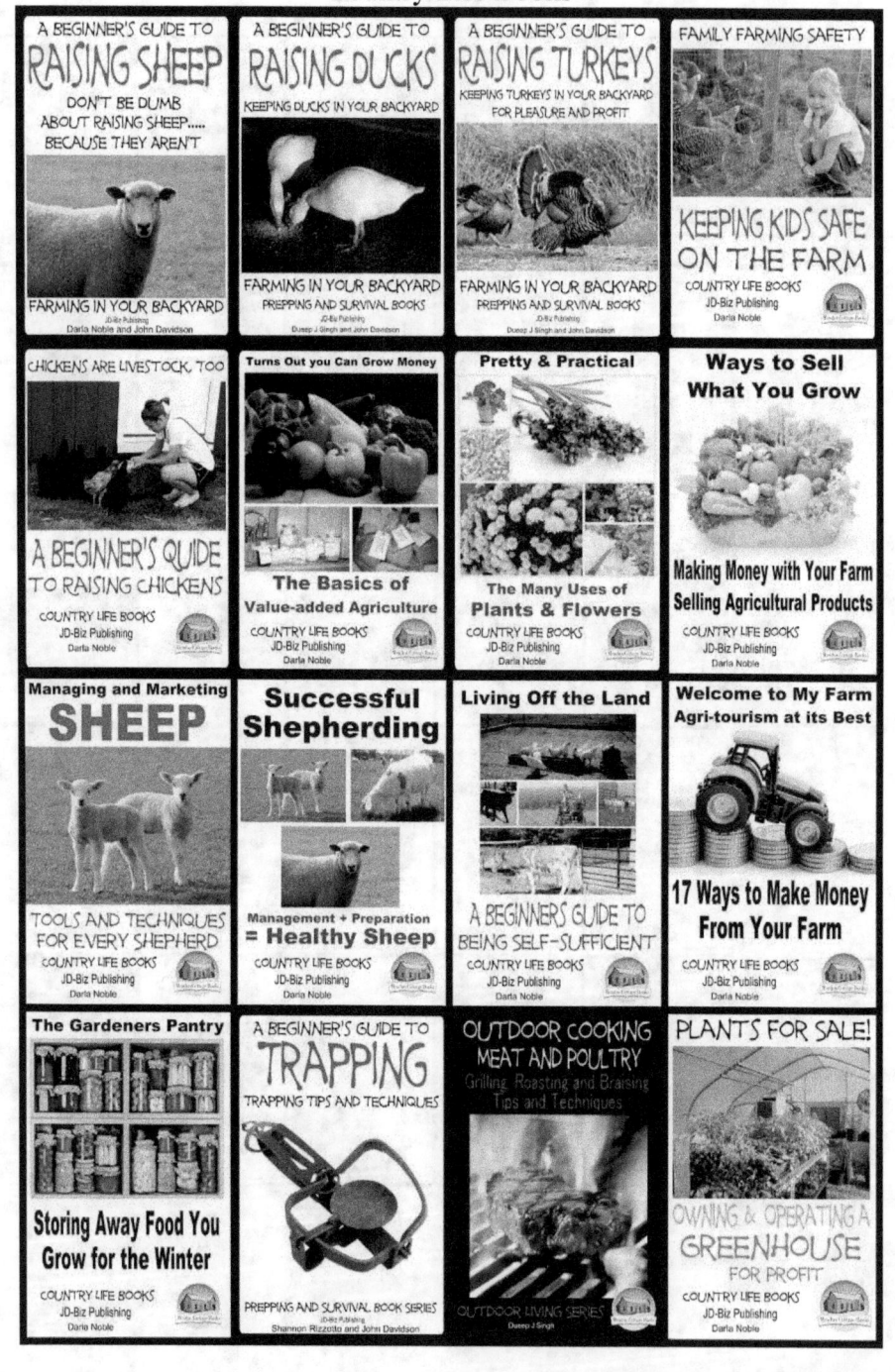

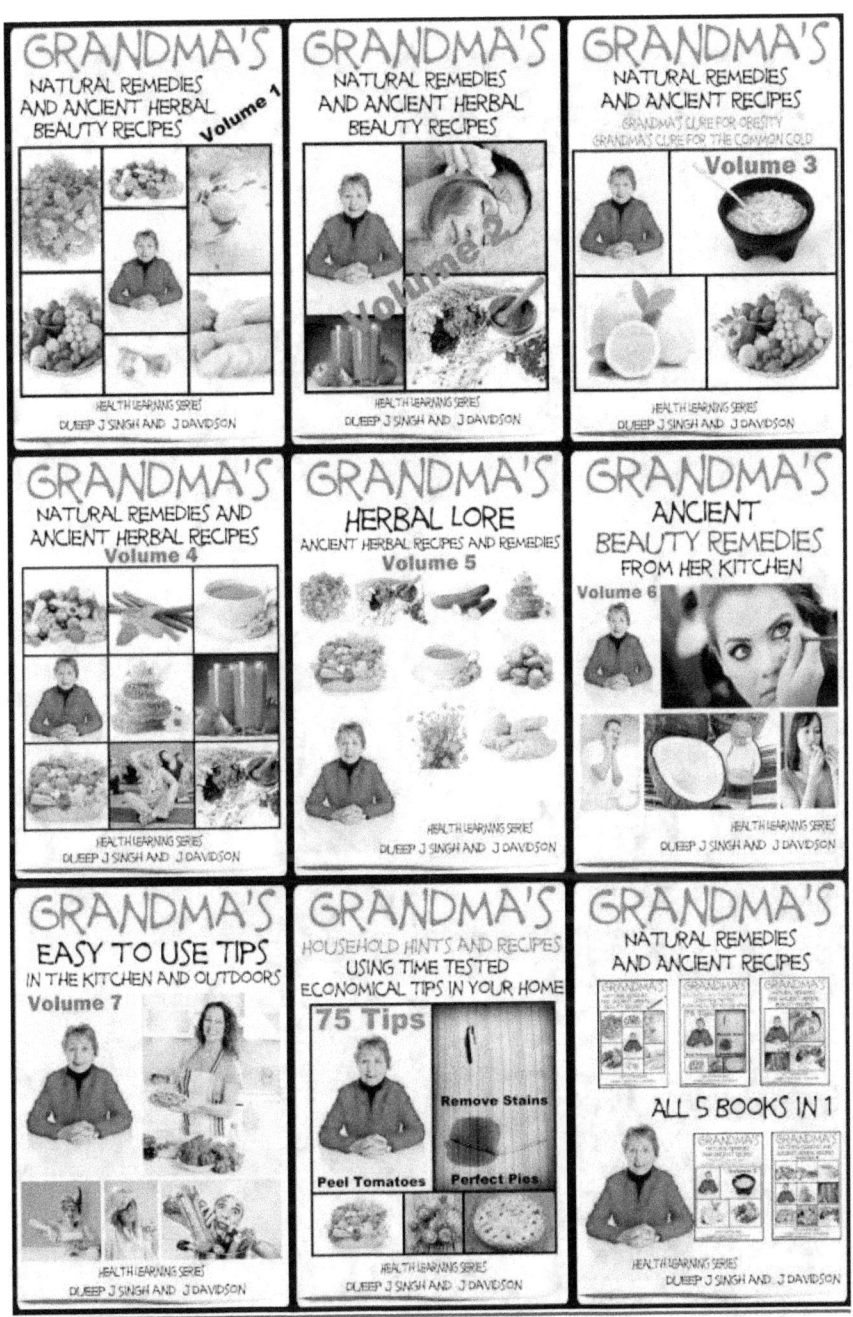

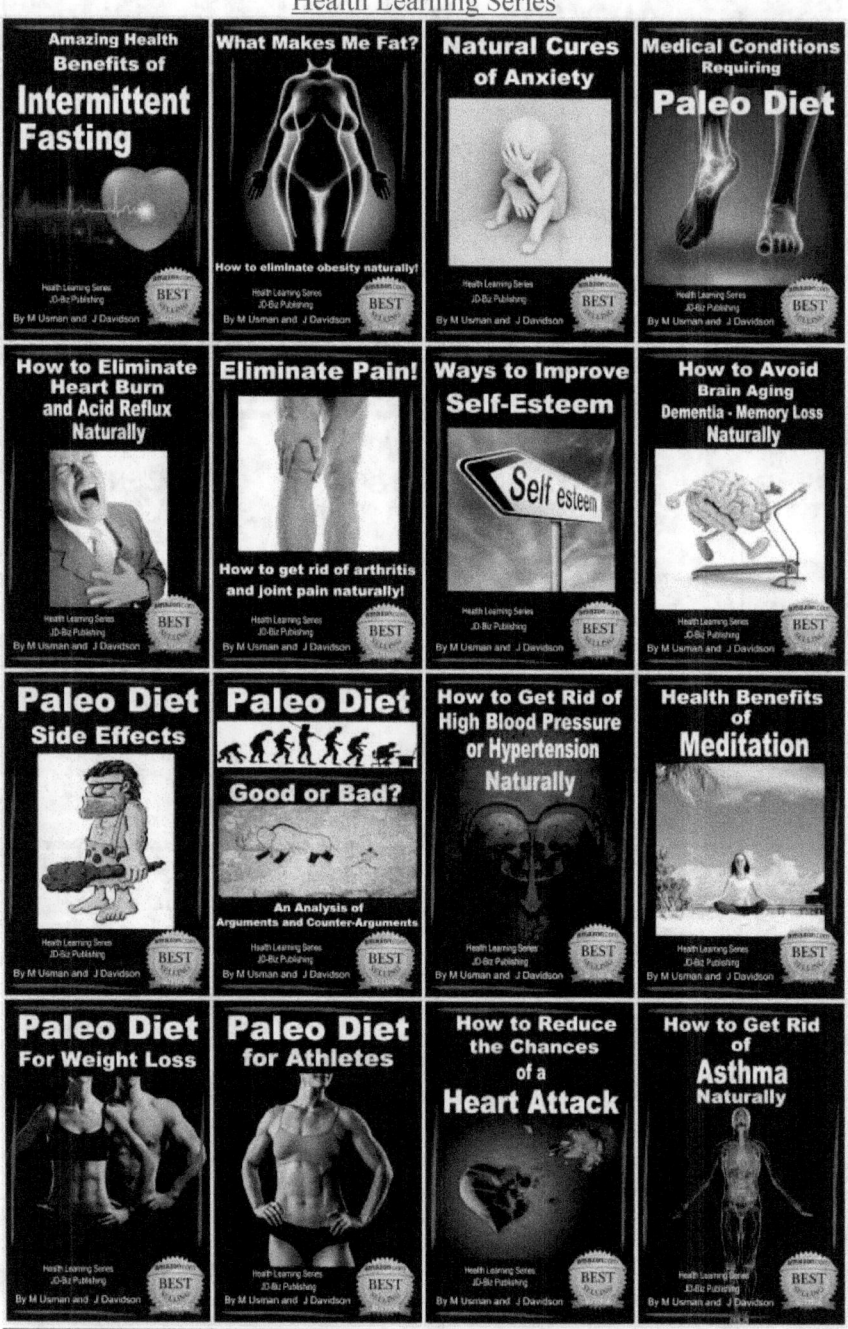

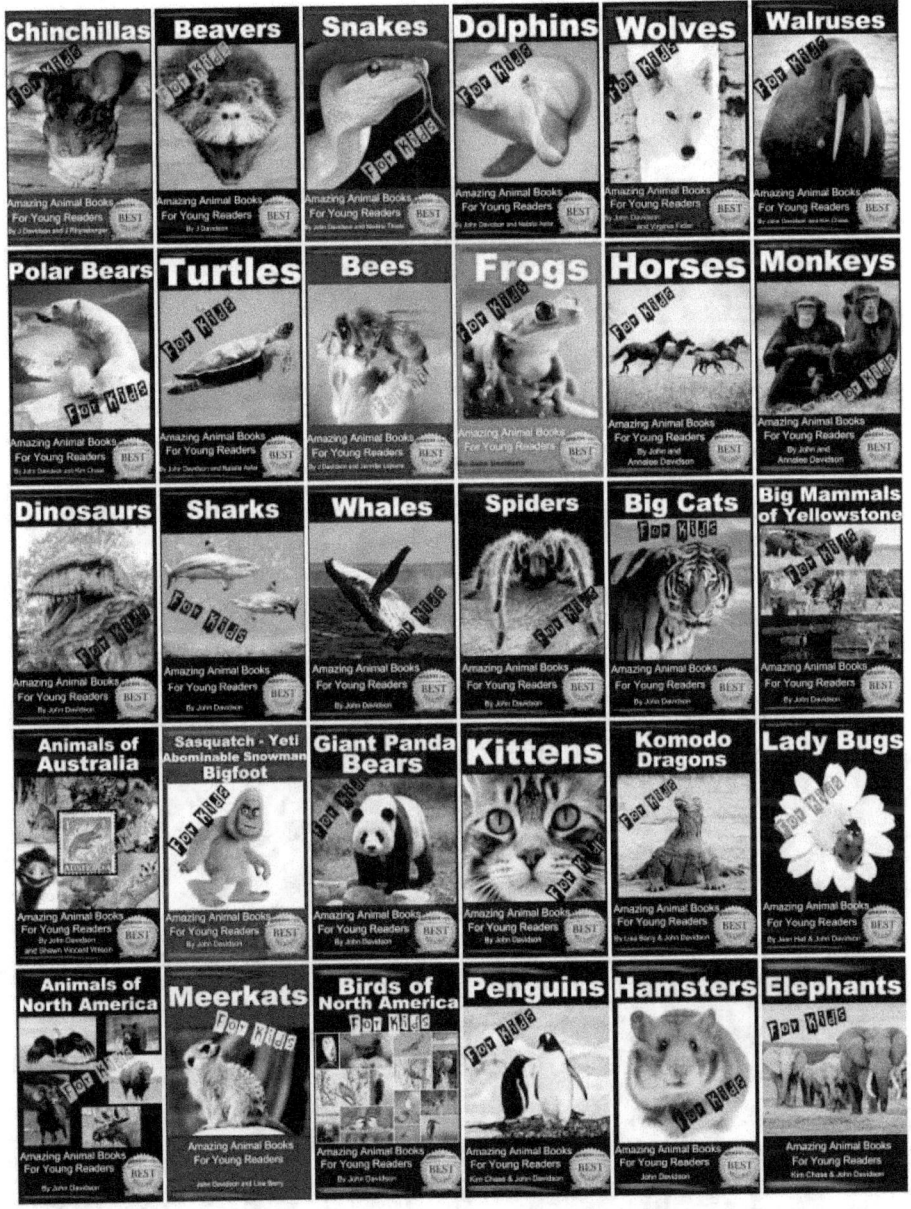

# Learn To Draw Series

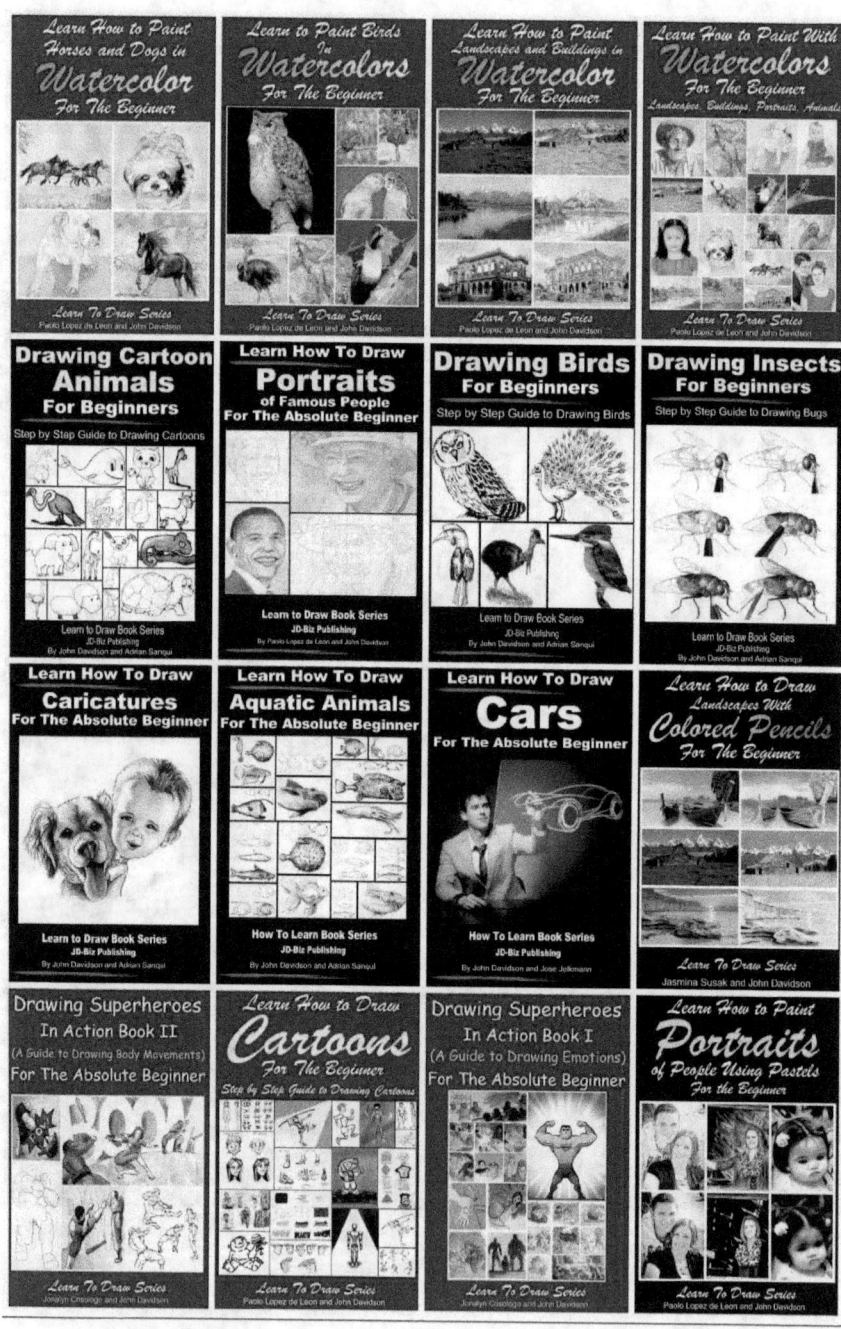

# How to Build and Plan Books

# Entrepreneur Book Series

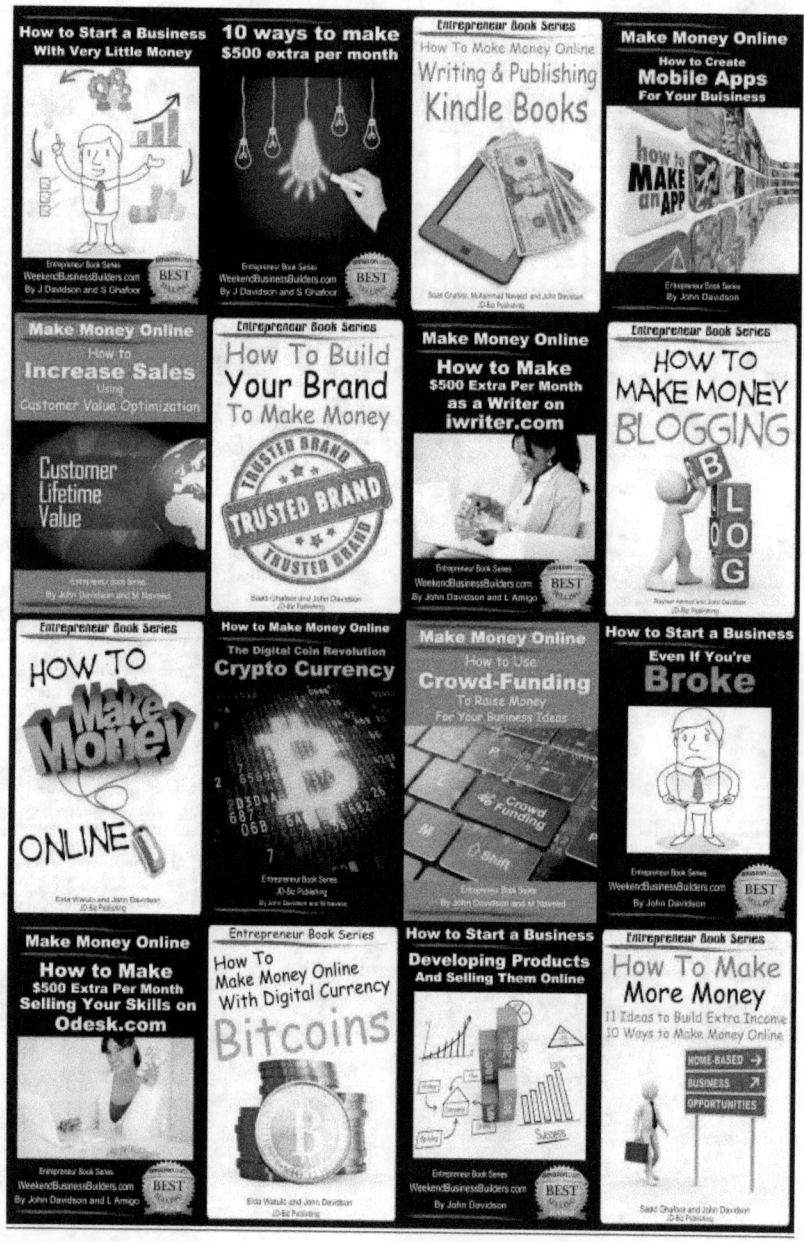

# Publisher

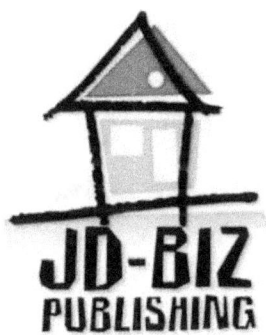

JD-Biz Corp

P O Box 374

Mendon, Utah 84325

http://www.jd-biz.com/

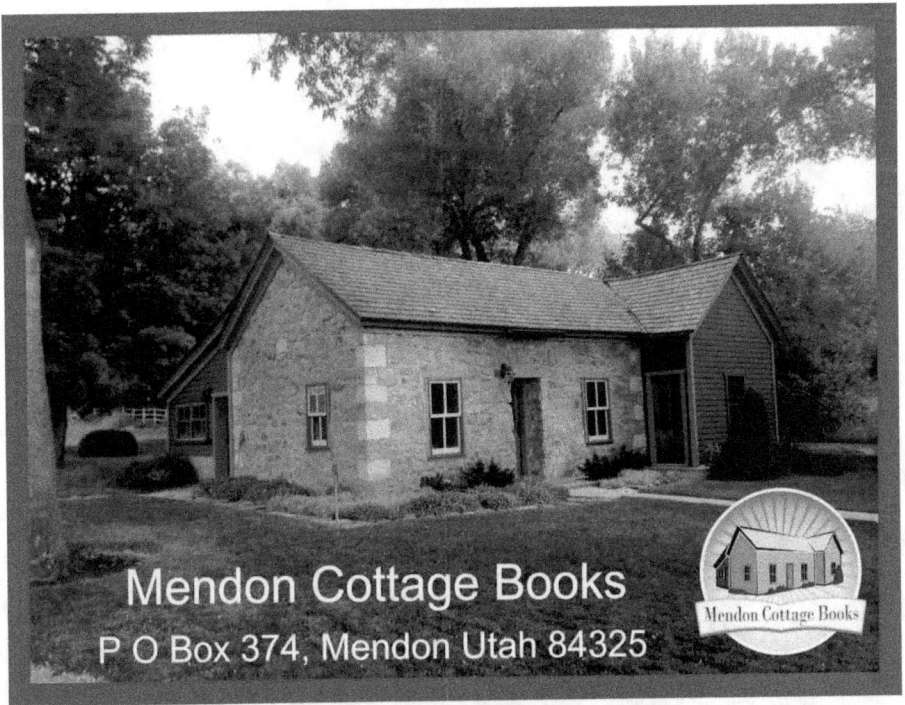

Mendon Cottage Books

P O Box 374, Mendon Utah 84325

www.ingramcontent.com/pod-product-compliance
Lightning Source LLC
Chambersburg PA
CBHW071137280526
45787CB00003B/1310